THE COMPLETE GUIDE TO PRIMITIVE EATING

David Soto Jr.

ISBN: 1508740186
ISBN-13: 978-1508740186

For my brother, Eric, a real life freakin' G.I. Joe, and his wife, Amy, who is also a bad ass. I mean, she's married to G.I. Joe.

TABLE OF CONTENTS

Preface..1

Introduction...4

Step 1: Dear Diary...8

Step 2: Know What You Are Eating.................12

Step 3: No More Sammiches...........................16

Step 4: Sharpen Your Skill-ets.....................19

Step 5: Stop Eating Breakfast.......................21

Step 6: Go Gluten-Free...................................24

Step 7: What A Crock.......................................30

Step 8: Go Legume Free.................................33

Step 9: Groceries, Groceries, Groceries.......37

Step 10: Go Dairy Free...................................39

Step 11: Educate Yourself..............................42

Step 12: Go Sugar Free..................................45

Step 13: Go Grain Free...................................50

Step 14: Go Grass Fed...................................54

Step 15: Go Chemical Free............................58

Chronic Inflammation and Disease............61
Closing Thoughts............................72

PREFACE

If you are coming here from my book, Mira!, I apologize for the repetition. The thing is, when I wrote Mira! I intended on repurposing the original content from the first version of the book you are now reading. When I started reusing the content, I saw the flaws in a lot of my writing and felt I had to dig deeper and do more research. I have also improved as a writer since writing this book back in 2013. I ended up with better content and felt it needed to go into a revised version. That's why some of the content you're about to read may seem familiar but that's ok. Repetition is the key to effective learning. Reading something once is often not enough. Reading and hearing information over and over again is very beneficial. That's why I made it Step 11 of this very program.

If you didn't come here from Mira!, disregard what you just read. I poured my heart and soul into this book just for you and would never think of repurposing content. (Wink, wink.) Honestly, Mira! was written for a very narrow audience who may have never come across the information found in this book, if I didn't write a book specifically for them. By the way, if you are a woman of Latin decent, I highly suggest you read Mira! I wrote it for you.

Don't forget this: The content in this book is not intended to be a substitute for professional medical advice, diagnosis, or treatment. Always seek the advice of your physician or other qualified health provider with any questions you may have regarding a medical condition. Never disregard professional medical advice or delay in seeking it because of something you have read in this book. Blah, blah, blah.

I am not a professional by any means. I do not have a college education, unless you count my Associates Degree from the Community College of the Air Force in Mechanical and Electrical Technology—which most people don't. I am not certified in anything. Nor do I have any letters in front of or after my name—unless Jr. counts. I am just an average guy who has read a lot of books, done a lot of research, and conducted a lot of experiments on himself. My goal is to take all this information and put it in the hands of other average people out there like me, with hopes of helping them reach their goal.

I truly hope you enjoy this book.

David Soto Jr., St. Louis, MO

INTRODUCTION

What is Primitive Eating?

Primitive Eating is eating food that has not been manipulated or made by man. Minimally processed or unprocessed food is what our bodies are designed to eat. Your body will accomplish amazing things when it does what it is designed to do, like eat natural, whole foods.

Something we may need to do here is draw the the line between what is processed and what is not. There are a lot of people who like to find fault like it's their job. They'll say that some Primitive foods are actually processed. This may have some truth to it but there is a minor detail that makes a significant difference. Almond butter, for example, is Primitive because it has one ingredient: almonds.

Yes, it is "processed" to actually make it into a nut butter but let's take that one ingredient and ask, can it be eaten whole and/or raw? The answer is, yes it can, and it commonly is. This is where that line is drawn. If something is inedible but is processed to make it "edible,' it is not Primitive. Wheat is the perfect example of this.

The typical "Primitive Eating" or "Paleo" challenge involves giving up grains, legumes, dairy, and added sugar for 30 days. The results are amazing and drastic. It works! No doubt about it. The problem is, the challenge is too hard for some people. Probably most people. So instead of pushing people to do a 30 day challenge, I thought, "What could people do to slowly transition into Primitive Eating?" That's when I came up with this idea: a self-paced step by step program.

My program is a combination of forming new habits and eliminating certain foods over a long period of time, at your own pace. This is a no-pressure method. If you get stuck at a step, keep working on it until you've mastered it. There is no timeline, so you won't fall behind. This is not a challenge so there is no chance of failing. Take your time. I do not recommend you do this with a partner or friend. The whole point is to go at your own pace and free yourself from any stress of trying compete or keep-up with anyone else.

How does the program work?

Once you get past this introduction, simply read the first step. Once you have met the requirements for mastering it, read the next step and move on. When you move on to step two, you will continue the new habit you have just learned in step one, and so on and so forth. You will continue this process until you reach the last step. Once at this point, you will have developed several life-changing habits, one at a time, at your own pace.

Note:
Since first publishing this book, I've found that most people have read the book cover to cover and then have gone back to start the program. This is not how I intended this book to work but who am I to complain about how people read my book. I am just grateful they are reading it!

Ready to get started?

STEP 1: DEAR DIARY

What to do:

Call it a food log, a food diary, or whatever you want but the point here is to start keeping track of what you eat. You can use your phone, a computer, or even a good ole' fashion note pad and pencil. It's your call. Be as vague or as detailed as you want. For example: "eggs and bacon," or "3 grade A large eggs, 4 slices uncured bacon from Trader Joe's." Make this as easy for yourself as possible. I do not want to make this a chore that you despise. This habit will be necessary in the future. Also, next to each meal note how you feel. Good, bad, tired etc. Example: "Eggs and bacon. — Satisfied." "Biscuits and gravy.— Bloated." "8oz Steak.— Energized and Happy."

Why do it:

This is a valuable habit to develop for two reasons:

1) Accountability! In my personal experience, and my experience as a personal trainer and weight loss coach, people tend to be much more responsible about what they eat when they have to write it down. Also, when other people have the potential to see what it is you are eating, you are going to be more cautious about what you consume. If you've ever used a budget for financing, you know what I am talking about. If you want to spend less money on useless crap, start writing down where you spend your money. Same goes for food!

2) You will have data to use for future reference. This is why writing how you feel is important. I got this idea when I noticed that I had been bloated for a couple of days. I had been keeping a food log but I did not keep track of how I felt. Had I, I would have been able to look back and see when I started feeling bloated to see what food may have been the culprit. In this particular case, I had to guess, it seemed like the bloating began when I started consuming two cloves of raw garlic a day. I cut out the garlic and the bloating subsided.

Also, after you have eliminated certain foods, you will be able to look back and see how much better you actually feel. This is going to be a huge motivator. You will actually be able to see when you stopped feeling tired or sluggish and see why, because these notes about how you feel will be right next to what it is you ate.

Note:

It is very important that you do not make any effort to change how you eat during the first two steps of this program. Developing these first two habits will prove very valuable in the future when you do start to make changes. The point here is to develop one new habit at a time. Ease into it.

When to move on:

When you have completed 7 consecutive days of food logging, move on to the next step. This is a daily habit. Continue logging your meals as you move on.

After some time you will be able to drop this habit. This is not something you will be required to do for the rest of your life. Within time, you will realize that you no longer need a food log for accountability.

STEP 2: KNOW WHAT YOU ARE EATING

What to do:

All you have to do in this step is know what you are eating. Again, no change in your eating habits is necessary. Just do not put anything in your mouth without knowing what it is first.

This should be an easy step but there will be some challenges. If you are eating a hardboiled egg with salt and pepper, the ingredients are clear. If you are dining out with friends, it may be a little more difficult.

But before we tackle the restaurant issue, let's cover a biggie: packaged foods. Packaged foods are required by law to have a label that lists their ingredients in order of predominance by weight. Simply put, the ingredients are listed in order from most prevalent to least. So before you eat that candy bar or microwavable meal, flip that sucker over and take a look at the ingredients. That's all. Read it, then eat it.

If you are at a restaurant, it's just a matter of being a little annoying. Here is a secret though: if you tell them you have a food allergy they will jump through hoops to provide you all the information you want.

Saying the following statement should get you all the information you need:

"I'm sorry to be a pain but I have a food allergy. Can you tell me how the ___ is prepared?"

If you are a person of integrity and don't want to lie, don't worry, you're not lying. You might have a food allergy or at least a sensitivity; you just don't know what it is yet.

Below are some questions I have asked that have yielded some strange looks from both friends and wait staff but prove to be effective.

- Is the salmon farm raised or wild caught?
- Where is your beef from?
- What kind of oil is it cooked in?
- Are your chicken wings breaded?
- Can I have your phone number?

Why do it:

1) INFORMATION! Just like the first step, you are gathering data. When you start realizing what it is you are actually putting in your body you may be less likely to do it. Again, I am not asking you to eliminate anything. You can still eat whatever you want. In fact, I want you to. I want you to see the crap you are putting in your body. Ignorance is bliss, but it is never, ever healthy!

2) Another reason for this habit is that the practice of reading labels and asking how your food is prepared will come in very handy when you start eliminating certain foods. It may not make sense right now but trust me, it will fall in place very soon.

When to move on:

Do this practice for seven days and then go on to the next step. This habit will never go away once it is set in place. Once you know there are certain things you do not want in your body, you will always read the label and never think twice about it. By now, you should have at least 14 days' worth of food log entries. That's some good data you've got there. Let's keep these two new habits up and move on to the next step.

STEP 3: NO MORE SAMMICHES

What to do:

Yep, here it is: your first elimination. Basically, kiss your sandwiches and burritos goodbye. In fact, kiss toast and rolls goodbye, too! That's right, you are giving up bread. I KNOW! I have heard it all before. I don't need to hear how much you love bread. I don't care. You are following this program because you have a goal in mind. This is a step towards that goal.

How do I do it? It's called a lettuce wrap. Many restaurants, like Five Guys, In-and Out, and Jimmy Johns, will wrap meat and cheese in lettuce at no extra cost. All you have to do is ask. If a place won't do it, just ask for it sans bun and eat it with fork. Or better yet, order a steak!

Why do it:

1) Later we are going to eliminate wheat. Consider this a baby step. Doing this will take a lot of stress off of going gluten-free. Chances are, you consume most of your wheat via bread. I'll go into more detail about how bad wheat is for you later when we get to the Gluten-Free step.

2) This is getting you out of the habit of eating on the run. Multitasking is overrated. Meals are meant to be enjoyed and eaten slowly. So settle down, get a knife and a fork, and eat.

3) If you are trying to lose weight, eliminating bread will make a significant difference in your body fat. This step alone will be a giant leap towards regulating your blood sugar levels and controlling your insulin spikes. Imagine eating a juicy ribeye with grilled veggies at your local steak house, but passing on the rolls. You will not only omit the rapid spike in insulin, (which causes your body to store fat) you will also avoid that bloated-and-then-tired feeling afterward. Not to mention, eliminating the large amount of calories you consume in bread alone. You will walk away from meals feeling just as satisfied but without having consumed all those extra, no purpose, calories.

When to move on:

When this is a part of your daily practice and you're feeling good, it's time to move on. Keep in mind, bread is out of your life. There are some recipes for "Primitive" bread out there but I don't recommend introducing them until much later.

STEP 4: SHARPEN YOUR SKILL-ETS

What to do:

This one is easy. Use a skillet to prepare one meal a day. That's it! Even if it's just to heat up left overs. If you really want to hone your skill-ets, use cast iron. Cast iron is the metal of choice for Primitive eaters. Nonstick pans may actually emit chemicals into the air you breathe when heated. Also, if you use a metal utensil when you cook, you could be scraping the nonstick coating into your food and that is not Primitive.

A well-seasoned cast iron pan, with a little help from some lard, can work just as good as nonstick skillets. Plus, you can put cast iron in the oven for roasting or baking. It's prefect for heating up leftovers.

Why do it:

This one may seem a little silly to some of us. The thing is, there are a lot of people out there who have a hard time eating Primitively because they don't know how to cook. They are so used to heating up prepackaged meals in a microwave or ordering out that cooking for themselves is out of the question. Well, in order to eat the Primitive way, you have to prepare your meals yourself. This habit is here for those of you who are culinarily challenged to get some practice in on the stove top!

When to move on:

When you have accomplished this task for 7 consecutive days you can move on. If you skip a day, you have to start over. Once you move past this step you don't have to keep it up for now, but you may find that it comes in handy in the future.

STEP 5: STOP EATING BREAKFAST

What to do:

No, I am not about to make you skip breakfast but you are about to skip the conventional breakfast food. In this step you will be learning that breakfast doesn't have to consist of your typical breakfast foods. Cereal, hash browns, pastries, and waffles are out. Anything else is in. So, get your cast iron skillet out and heat up last night's left overs because you are not having breakfast for breakfast for a while.

Why do it:

1) Chances are your current breakfast habits are killing you. Consuming sugar and things that turn into sugar first thing in the morning is detrimental to your health. These "meals" will raise your blood sugar, drain your energy, and make you hungry again within just a few hours. Is this really how you want to start your day?

2) The next step after this is a biggie, and now that you have eliminated bread, the next step is to eliminate your typical breakfast foods. Accomplishing these two steps is going to make the next one that much easier.

3) Who determined that only certain foods can be eaten in the morning? For all we know, it was processed food manufacturers who needed to develop a market for their products. Supposedly, normal people eat cereal for breakfast, but guess what? Normal people are sick and obese. Be weird! Be healthy! Eat leftover ribs for breakfast.

When to move on:

When you have done this habit for 7 days in a row, you can move on. You can resume eating breakfast foods but you are going to find that as you move on to the next step you are going to be very limited with what you can eat for breakfast. I have two words for you: Bacon and Eggs.

STEP 6: GO GLUTEN-FREE

What to do:

This is it folks. This is your first really big challenge. Going gluten-free is not easy but the rewards are incredible. From now on, consider yourself gluten-free. This means no wheat, rye, or barley products. Bread, tortillas, cereals, pancakes, and waffles are already out of your diet. Those were all stepping stones to this step. Now, you have to cut out the pasta and sweets made with flour.

Oh, and remember all that practice you got reading labels? Well now it's time to put those skills to good use. Start looking for gluten in your food that isn't an obvious wheat product. Here are two good examples: I thought soy sauce, of all things, would be gluten free. I mean, it's SOY sauce for Pete's sake. One day I took a look at the label and, lo and behold, there it was, plain as day: WHEAT. (If you're looking for a gluten-free soy sauce, try Tamari or, even better, coconut aminos.) Here's the other example: after months of feeling bad, someone suggested that I try to go gluten-free. Well, I thought had been gluten-free for over two years by this time but this person said that I had the symptoms of someone who was having a negative reaction to gluten. I thought, "Impossible. I know what I eat." The only thing I didn't know for sure was my supplements. When I checked my B complex vitamin, can you guess what I found? WHEAT.

In the future you will not be eating anything labeled "Gluten-free." Anything labeled as such is usually processed junk, BUT if it is going to make your transition a little easier, I will allow some "Gluten-free" products. Just remember your goal is to eat Primitive. Gluten-free doughnuts are not Primitive. Also, if you are trying to drop some excess pounds of fat, keep in mind that the wheat flour substitutes commonly found in Gluten-free products will cause you to store fat nearly as much as wheat flour will. Brown rice flour may not have all the side effects as wheat flour, but it has one: It makes you fat. That's a pretty important side effect. Be wary of anything labeled "Gluten-free!" Eat a steak instead.

Cross contamination is something to look out for. Take this example: You find out your favorite chicken wing joint has a food allergy menu online. You check it out and find that most of their flavored wings are actually gluten-free. Great, right? Let's go down to have a cider and some hot wings. The problem is, this place fries their wings in the same oil they fry their onion rings, breaded chicken strips, and boneless wings in (which are also breaded). Sad news friend, your wings are not gluten-free. Know what you are eating!

Why do it:

1) Whether it is whole or raw, wheat is inedible. A kernel of wheat is made of three parts: The bran, the germ, and the endosperm. The endosperm is the pretty white part we make into bread. It is also the reproductive part of the plant. Like all living things, this plant wants to reproduce. So to protect its young, it covers the endosperm with the bran. The bran is indigestible so even if the kernel is eaten, it will pass through the digestive tract intact. If it were to get pooped out in dirt, let's say, you would have yourself a nearly perfect condition for this plant to grow.

What we do as humans is separate the endosperm, the "edible" part, by processing it. We turn it into flour and then turn the flour in to things like, tortillas, bread, and pasta. What we are essentially doing is consuming something we would not be able to consume in nature and doing it in LARGE quantities.

2) You could be allergic. Yeah, yeah, I know what you are thinking. "I am not allergic" or "I don't have celiac disease." I believe we are all react negatively to wheat in some way. Some of us more than others. And just because you test negative for celiac doesn't mean that test was accurate. The majority of the tests out there are inaccurate. Thus, people are being sent home from the doctor's office after being told they are not allergic, so they can, and do, continue to eat wheat. They also stay sick.

Your body doesn't see wheat as food (because it is not). It sees it as bacteria, so your white blood cells attack it. This causes inflammation, a swelling in your gut that Dr. William Davis calls "Wheat Belly." I have seen one of my client's waistlines shrink inches in just 30 days, but he had only lost five pounds. Why the drastic loss of inches but not a drastic loss in weight? He gave up wheat and the swelling simply went down.

3) It's addictive. I know someone who is sick. All of her symptoms are signs of gluten intolerance. She has been sick for years and has seen several doctors during this time. She was frustrated and tired of feeling ill. I told her that all she had to do was go gluten-free. She tried it but found it to be difficult. She found that if she just ate a little bit she actually felt better. That, folks, is called withdrawal. Gliadin, gluten's buddy present in wheat and other grains, has been said to have an opiate effect on the brain. When you give it up abruptly you may experience withdrawal. If your body throws a fit because it has to go without something it's used to, that is an addiction. Generally speaking, if something is addictive, it's not good for you. Am I right? Cigarettes, crack, sugar, heroin, booze? There is no health benefit to consuming gluten. It just makes you want to eat more stuff that will make you sick.

4) Wheat raises you blood sugar higher than... SUGAR! Have you heard of the Glycemic Index? The Glycemic Index is used to measure how much specific foods increase you blood sugar levels, otherwise known as blood glucose. Depending on which chart you look at, white bread will be higher than whole wheat or vice versa, but on most charts you will see that both are actually higher than table sugar! Yet the government recommends a diet rich in whole grains. Doesn't make sense, does it?

When to move on:

This could be, by far, the hardest step you are going to have to get through but the benefits are going to be the greatest. This step will also take you the longest to get a hold of. Don't be surprised if this takes a month. When this habit seems like second nature and you are past any withdrawal stages, it's time to move on to the next step.

STEP 7: WHAT A CROCK

What to do:

Don't have enough time to cook? Take longer to do it!

If you don't have a crock pot, get one. This manner of cooking is a time saver. An old friend of mine hated the concept of cooking with a crock pot until I moved in and brought mine with me. Now she uses it at least once a week, specifically on the nights when she won't have time to make dinner.

Personally, I am no expert on crock pot cooking but I will teach you what I know:

1) Put in a chunk of meat; pot roast, pork shoulder, etc.
2) Throw in whole spices; garlic, pepper corns, bay leaf, etc.
3) Put it on a low setting
4) 8 hours later, eat it!

It's that easy.

Things to keep in mind:

- You will usually have a ton of left overs so plan accordingly. I once made several pounds of pork shoulder and topped it all with a chili verde salsa. Guess what I got tired of eating after a week or so? Since, I have learned to make different sauces on the side. So yeah, I may be eating pork for a few days in a row but every night is a different flavor.
- You can use your crock pot to make bone broth (Just follow the instructions above, except replace the chunk of meat with bones. Oh, and add water and bit of apple cider vinegar).

- Get the kind of crock pot where you can remove the ceramic part of the pot. It will be easier to clean.

Why do it:

It's super easy. That's pretty much it. Not a chef? Perfect! This method of cooking requires very little, if any, culinary skills.

When to move on:

After three crock pot meals you are ready to move on.

STEP 8: GO LEGUME FREE

What to do:

Legumes are your next elimination. That means, beans or anything that comes in a pod. So (are you ready for this?), this includes peanuts. They may be labeled as nuts, but they are NOT. Pinto beans, lentils, black beans, garbanzo beans, and soy beans, are all included in what you are giving up, but keep in mind that products made from these items are also on the list. This will include: hummus, peanut butter, soy sauce, chocolate, and certain vegetable oils.

Why do it:

Let's look at some of the drawbacks to eating legumes:

- Lectins. Lectins are one of the things that can damage the lining of the small intestine. That being said, one of the main reasons for omitting all of the foods I am suggesting you eliminate is to allow your gut to heal.
- Phytic acid. This prevents any nutrients that legumes may have from actually being absorbed by the body.
- FODMAPs. FODMAP stands for Fermentable Oligosaccharides, Disaccharides, Monosaccharides And Polyols which are a cause of major IBS symptoms such as gas, pain, and diarrhea. Remember the old playground tune: "Beans, Beans, They're good for you heart. The more you eat the more you fart?"

Soy is the number-one genetically modified organism (GMO) in the U.S. It is basically created in a lab and mass produced in the fields. This is not food. Not even close. When you eat soy you are eating something that cannot be found in nature.

This alone is enough reason for me not to eat soy but let's look a little further into it.

In addition to the drawbacks listed above, soy contains a high concentration of phytoestrogens. Phytoestrogens act as estrogen in the body. The overconsumption of soy can lead to what is know as Estrogen Dominance or Estrogen Toxicity.

I am certainly no expert in the area of estrogen but a little research on the internet yielded this long list of estrogen toxicity symptoms.

- Breast tenderness
- Depression, fatigue, poor concentration
- Endometriosis
- Fibrocystic breast
- PMS
- Fibroids
- Water retention and bloating
- Fat gain around hips and thighs
- Breast and uterine cancer
- Difficultly losing weight
- Infertility
- Irregular menstrual periods
- Low sex drive, low libido

All good reasons not to eat soy, no?

Believe it or not, I was once a vegetarian. In attempt to increase my protein intake, I started drinking protein shakes made with soy protein. This essentially, uh… took the lead out of my pencil, if you know what I mean. After a couple weeks, and a little research, I stopped with the soy protein shakes and almost immediately got my manhood back. I gladly threw the rest of my soy protein powder in the trash and never looked back.

When to move on:

When you get the hang of this one, feel free to move on.

STEP 9: GROCERIES, GROCERIES, GROCERIES

What to do:

Buy groceries at least three times a week. And, try to hit other sources other than your mega grocery store. Try farmers markets, local farmers, mom and pop grocers, and butchers.

Why do it:

1) You are eating fresher food with fewer or no preservatives. Because of this, food tends to go bad sooner. Buying a week's worth of food at one time will no longer work.

2) It gives you the freedom to eat what you feel like eating. If you have ground beef that has been sitting in the fridge for a few days but you want chicken, too bad; that beef needs to be cooked. But if you have an empty fridge and want to grill some boneless, skinless chicken thighs, all you have to do is run in and grab a pound or two.

3) You will actually spend less time. If you are on your way home and need to get dinner started, you don't have time to grab a cart and walk up and down each isle. You'll need to get in there, get what you need, and get out. This will save you a ton of time.

4) You will save a bunch of money. Buying nutrient dense food isn't cheap but they're FULL of nutrients. So you eat less, and in turn, buy less. Also, since you are buying fewer and fewer foods with long shelf lives to be stored in your cabinets, you are also spending less.

When to move on:

When you get two weeks of three or more grocery trips per week, it will be time to move on.

STEP 10: GO DAIRY FREE

What to do:

Here is another toughie. Up until now you have probably been enjoying milk, ice cream, and more likely than anything else, CHEESE. It's time to let it go. From this point forward, you are now dairy free.

Why do it:

I like to base everything I talk about on what comes most natural to us as humans. Does drinking milk from another animal's breast seem natural? Think about it. Why would one species drink the milk created by another species? Whale's milk is made for whales. Dog's milk is made for dogs.

Human's milk is made for humans. And cow's milk is made for cows.

The milk we buy in the store is pasteurized and homogenized. Most of the nutrients in it are destroyed in these processes. Also, the chemical structure of the milk is changed when it is pasteurized and homogenized. It's basically not even milk anymore. It's as un-natural as can be by the time it gets to your refrigerator.

Dairy is an irritant that can lead to chronic inflammation and autoimmune disorders (I cover this later in this book). Personally, too much dairy leads to excess mucus production, upset stomach, and acne. Let's look at the two ingredients in milk that contribute to all of these symptoms, lactose and casein.

Lactose

Most of us can't digest lactose. We stop producing the enzyme that helps digest it soon after infancy. It makes sense, doesn't it? This would be about the time we would have been weaned off of our mother's breast.

Words that end in "-ose" indicate that they are a sugar. Eg. Fructose, glucose, and sucrose. The word lactose simply means, milk sugar. I cover the negative effects of sugar later in this book.

Casein

The milk protein, casein, has been linked to autism and type one diabetes. These two diseases are formed in infancy. Do you understand this? The very thing you are giving your children could be the cause of two life long conditions.

Casein has an opiate effect thanks to casomorphins. Guess where there is a high concentration of casein? CHEESE! This is may be why people just flat out refuse to give up cheese.

When to move on:

After 14 days of going dairy-free, you are ready to move on. You will probably feel a lot better and even look a bit slimmer.

STEP 11: EDUCATE YOURSELF

What to do:

Read an article, a blog post, chapter of a book or listen to a podcast by one of the following:

- Robb Wolf
- Chris Kresser
- Mark Sisson
- Diane Sanfilippo
- Shawn Stevenson

I consider all of these people to be Primitive eating gurus and I have personally reached out to a couple of them for advice. There are many more people out there but the blogs, podcasts, and books written by these geniuses are responsible for the majority of my knowledge on this subject.

Why do it:

1) Knowledge is Power! The more informed you get about your health the more you are going to be willing to make the necessary changes.

2) Repetition is Key. Some of the things you are going to hear or read are going to seem odd or contrary to what you have been told your whole life. You may be resistant to some of these ideas. But, when you start hearing them over and over again, from credible sources, you are going to eventually start to believe them instead of the bad information you have been fed all these years.

3) Motivation. My close friend, Zig Ziglar, (we've actually never met) said, "People often say that motivation doesn't last. Well, neither does bathing, that's why we recommend both, daily." When you start reading or listening, you are going to come across stories or testimonials of people who have had symptoms similar to yours and how their symptoms disappeared after eliminating something for just a couple of weeks. Listening to these stories is going to give you hope and it'll motivate you to keep going. I know it does for me.

When to move on:

When you have done this habit for 7 consecutive days you will be ready and motivated to tackle your next habit. And, trust me, you are going to need all the motivation you can get.

STEP 12: GO SUGAR FREE

What to do:

This one is going to hurt, but it's time to go sugar free. And yeah, I mean all sugars and even artificial sweeteners. Table sugar, honey, maple syrup, agave nectar, stevia, equal, and basically any ingredient that ends in "ose." Those "gluten-free" treats, like cookies, they go bye-bye. Take note, that I am not saying "carbs." I am saying SUGAR.

Also, I know you're not going to like this, but fruit is including in this step. Fruit would be an occasional treat to a hunter-gatherer. Don't believe me? Go outside right now and find some wild fruit to pick! Fruit is seasonal and geographical. To have a variety of fruit from different parts of the world at our fingertips is not something our body is designed to handle.

Why do it:

I cover the negative effects of sugar extensively in the diabetes section of this book so, what I want to do here is take a common sense look at how unnatural it is for us to eat sugar.

How much sugar do you think our ancestors had access too?

Every living creature has one goal and that is to produce a surviving offspring. This includes plants. Some plants protect their seeds by covering it with and indigestible coating, such as wheat. Others protect it with bio-toxins, such as potatoes and tomatoes. Some use the flavor of bitterness as a warning not to eat them. In the case of fruit, like berries, it's the opposite. They want to be eaten so they can be passed through the digestive system a dropped at another location to sprout and grow. This is why berries are bright in color and sweet.

When it comes to foraging for food out in the wild, when something is bitter it is a good indication not to eat it. However if something is sweet, your body instinctually gives the green light to eat it. You see, sugar is not easily found in nature. Your body knows this, so when you introduce something sweet to your body, it goes nuts. Your body says, eat as much of this while you can.

This point was really made clear to me when I watched Out of the Wild — Venezuela. In this show 9 strangers were dropped in the middle of nowhere and had to walk out, over 70 miles, with limited supplies and no food. After just a couple days, they were starving. But unlike other survival shows, they didn't just have to survive for a few days and wait to be rescued, they had to walk out. A few quit but the rest pressed on, killing a foraging whatever they could in order to eat. The scene I remember the most, like I was there myself, was the one where they were walking one day and stumbled across a patch of wild blueberries. Like animals, they dropped to their knees and went crazy picking and eating the berries.

I can't think of a better example of our human survival instincts kicking in. Their body told them to "eat as much as you can." Why? 1) They were mobile. They needed the energy to continue to walk. Also, because they were walking to safety, this meant they had to eventually leave the berry patch. They had to fill up and go. 2) The berries were a rare find. They had gone days without seeing any. Who knows when they would see another patch. 3) The berries were sweet. This let them know they were safe to eat.

This isn't a theory on how our ancestors reacted to sugar. This is a real life accounting of how humans reacted to sugar, in 2010.

Now, imagine this instinctive reaction to sugar when you are at a restaurant, your home, or the grocery store! Sugar is not so hard to find now. The grocery store is full of isle upon isle of it. Your cupboards are full of it too. It is so available that you don't even have to chew to get it. You can just pour it into your body in the form of juices, soda, and caramel lattes. How are are you supposed to turn off this instinct to "eat as much as you can?" In the wild you didn't have to. You would either leave where the sugar was available or you would simply run out. But, in this day and age, these two scenarios are nearly impossible.

Have you ever been to a Native American reservation? If you have, you may have noticed a syringe disposal container in **every** public bathroom. This is an indicator of how common diabetes is among indigenous people. This is what happens when you introduce sugar into a community of hunter-gatherers.

When to move on:

Move on to the next step when you are sugar free for 21 days. If you want, after your 21 days, you can incorporate some fruit. But if you are trying to lose weight, you may want to stay away until you lean out.

STEP 13: GO GRAIN FREE

What to do:

By now you are probably still eating rice, corn and (if you are weird), quinoa. Well, now it's time to get rid of them. If you are like me when I started this, you might be thinking, "Corn is a grain?" We have been taught that it is a "vegetable" but it's NOT! It is a grain.

Here are just some of the things you may still be eating but will now be giving up: Any gluten-free treats made with brown rice flour, corn tortillas, rice cakes, tortilla chips, rice krispies, corn flakes, oatmeal, popcorn, corn bread, quinoa, and amaranth.

Why do it:

In 1956 the U.S. Government started recommending the Four Basic Food Groups. They were, fruits and vegetables, dairy, meat, and grains. Depending on your age, you may remember this being taught to us in elementary school. In 1992 the U.S. implemented the Food Pyramid. At the base of the Food Pyramid, the largest portion, was the recommendation of 6-11 servings of grains, cereal, bread, and pasta. Though there was a slight change to the Food Pyramid in 2005, it held strong until 2011 when it was replaced with My Plate. My Plate is essentially a pie chart depicting that 30% of your plate should contain grains. For 60 years the U.S. Government has been programing us to eat grains. No wonder so many people have issues with being told not to eat them. Guess which branch of the government is responsible with putting out all of this information over the past 6 decades? The U.S. Department of AGRICULTURE!

Corn is not food and, as a result, it wreaks havoc on your gut. I know this is a bold statement but let's go back to the end of WWII. A surplus of

Ammonium Nitrate, that was manufactured for munitions, was repurposed as fertilizer. This fertilizer supplied the corn with it's much needed nitrogen and farmers could now grow corn season after season. And, because corn was more profitable due to government subsidies, they did.

What you have to realize here is the the nitrogen supplied by Ammonium Nitrate is synthetic, man made. The natural process the involves the sun was replaced with a chemical process that used natural gas instead, essentially making corn petroleum based. Take this and the fact that corn has been genetically modified to produce a higher yield, resist pesticides, or even produce their own pesticide makes corn completely unnatural and thus, no longer food. Remember how I said soy was the number one genetically modified organism? Well, corn is number two!

Do you know what ranchers feed cattle to make them fat? GRAINS! They feed them grains for this specific reason. It makes them fat and it will do the same to you! This realization alone was enough for me to give up grains. No science needed here. Not for me anyway!

When to move on:

After 14 days of being grain free you should be ready to move on. Oh, and by the way, if you have completed this step, you're pretty much a Primitive eater. There are two more steps but these two will bump you up to super elite status and may be dependent on your budget.

STEP 14: GO GRASS FED

What to do:

If you are a meat eater, you probably eat a lot of beef. Well, in this step you are going to start incorporating grass fed beef into your diet. In just the past couple of years grass fed beef has gone from being only found in Whole Foods and Trader Joe's to being found at your local super market, Aldi and even Target. You can find a pound of ground grass fed beef anywhere from $6.99 to $8.99.

I want you to consider pastured and wild meats as well. Any animal that is free to live its life walking around outside is going to be a better choice than those that are raised in confined spaces indoors, never seeing the light of day their entire life.

Why do it:

You shouldn't eat grains and neither should your food!

Please note the quote below from PubMed.gov.

"Excessive amounts of omega-6 polyunsaturated fatty acids (PUFA) and a very high omega-6/omega-3 ratio, as is found in today's Western diets, promote the pathogenesis of many diseases, including cardiovascular disease, cancer, and inflammatory and autoimmune diseases, whereas increased levels of omega-3 PUFA (a low omega-6/omega-3 ratio) exert suppressive effects."

What most people don't know is that they are eating too many foods high in omega-6 fatty acids. Omega-6 is found in commercially raised and grain fed animals. Beef, pork, chicken, and fish that are not wild caught or pastured are throwing off your omega-6 to omega-3 ratio.

One thing that sticks out to me is how good people feel when they start a juice cleanse or a vegetarian diet. The reason the feel so good could actually be because they are drastically eliminating the amount of omega-6 they are consuming. These initial results are only temporary though, which is why this is not a book on the vegetarian diet.

One of the best way to improve our omega-6/omega-3 ratio is by simply replacing the animal fat you consume, that's high omega-6, with those high in omega-3. This is done my eating pasture raised or wild caught meat, fish, fowl, and eggs. Yes, replacing farm raised salmon with wild caught salmon means you are consuming fats high in omega-3 rather than omega-6. How can the same animal produce difference qualities of fat? Simple, one is fed GRAINS.

Cows that eat grass are out in the pasture walking around and enjoying life. Cows raised in stock yards eat grains and are usually knee deep in mud and shit. This may cause them to get sick, so as a preventative measure, they are given antibiotics. Also, they may or may not be given growth hormones and god knows what else. I knew a guy who raised cows and fed them ground up expired breakfast cereal, box and all! All of this is makes the cows fat, tasty and profitable. The problem is that fat stores toxins! When you eat the tasty animal fat in that ribeye you may be also consuming the toxins that the cow was fed or exposed to.

Animal fat is good for you but only when that animal eats Primitive, like you!

When to move on:

By now you are a pretty healthy person and the only thing that could possibly hold you back from this habit is the cost. If you have a freezer full of meat, you do not have to throw it all away because you are on this step. Just start slowly stocking up on grass fed beef. Move on to the final step whenever you are ready.

STEP 15: GO CHEMICAL FREE

What to do:

Now it's time to start implementing some organic vegetables into your life. Especially with vegetables you do not have to peel to eat. Also, you already read labels but now it's time to look at the ones on your bathroom and cosmetic products.

A simple way to look at this is if you can't pronounce it, don't use/eat it. Or, if you can pronounce it but don't know what the hell it is, don't use/eat it. This statement has now been elevated to the level of "controversy" as of late. There has been a lot of hubbub on the internet in attempt to debunk this but it's B.S. I'll explain.

According to the rule mentioned above, would you eat something if you found the following in its ingredients list: proline, methionine, or cystine? The obvious answer to this is, no. This question is a trick, meant to make people look stupid. Proline, methionine, and cystine are amino acids found in a banana. This is where people on the internet virtually point at you and say with a sense of satisfaction, "Ha! According to your rule you can eat it!" Here is the thing, if an ingredient is naturally found in a food it is not required to be added to the food label. This is why the sticker on a banana only says, banana. If something is used to make the food, it is required to be on the label, even if it's water. Do you see the difference?

Why do it:

You already don't eat crap. So why would you apply crap to your skin, your body's largest organ! There is no such thing as "for external use only." Your body absorbs everything that comes in contact with your skin. The illusion that you will be safe as long as something doesn't go "in" your body is false.

Why do you think dermal prescription patches work? A rule of thumb, albeit a tough one, is to not put anything on your skin that you would not put in your mouth.

I hate to do this to you but here is a list of things you are going to have to either find an alternate for or eliminate all together:

- Antiperspirant/Deodorant
- Soap
- Lotion
- Shampoo
- Conditioner
- Sun Screen
- Toothpaste
- Make up

When to move on:

This is the last step. There is no moving on. Slowly work on incorporating this last step and don't forget to enjoy your life!

CHRONIC INFLAMMATION AND DISEASE

Inflammation is your body's way of healing itself.
There are two types: Acute and Chronic

Acute Inflammation

You have more than likely experienced acute
inflammation when you sprained your ankle or got
stung by a bee. The result is the affected area can
become swollen, red, painful, or even warm.
Typically these affects go away over a short period
of time, when the threat is gone. If the inflammation
persist, it is a good indication that something more
serious is actually wrong. People who thought their
wrist was sprained often find out it is actually broken

after the swelling does not go away after a couple days.

Chronic Inflammation

Chronic inflammation effects your body the same way as acute inflammation (pain, swelling, redness, and heat) but is present over a long duration of time, months or even YEARS. Imagine your body's reaction to a bee sting never going away. Now imagine this bee sting happening inside your body where it is kind of hidden. (It's not hidden for a lot of you but more on this later.)

Now, what causes chronic inflammation? There is a lot of science out there that answers this question and I'm not going got lie, some of it is way over my head. Let me try and break it down for you.

1) Chronic inflammation can be a result of an autoimmune response or disorder. This is when your immune system attacks healthy tissue, mistaking it for infectious agents. Examples of this are: Crohn's disease, celiac disease, and irritable bowel syndrome. Now, what causes this response? Intestinal permeability. Intestinal permeability is

basically holes in the protective lining of your intestinal tract. These holes allow, well, shit to leak out of your gut and into the rest of your body. Hint: Shit is not supposed to be anywhere but your intestine!

What causes these holes in your gut? Well, the most common answer I have found in my research is Gliadin, which is found in wheat. Other foods that have evidence of causing leaky gut are, can you guess, grains, legumes (like peanuts and soy), and sugar. Stress and medications are also well known contributors.

2) The other cause for chronic inflammation is a steady, low intensity irritant. This is the real killer. It's doing people harm and they don't even know it. So for those people who are like, I don't have Crohn's disease or I was tested for Celiac and I don't have it, they are worse off. Because they are not diagnosed with a disease, they feel they are free to eat cake or whatever and, as a result, they maintain a low level of inflammation over years or even decades.

Note:

I want to point out that to you. If you consider your immune system an army, and you have an autoimmune disorder, your soldiers are constantly in a war. A war that doesn't exist. If all your soldiers are busy fighting a war, what happens when there is a real invader? You get sick. Ever wonder why some people are never sick and some people seem to always get sick? We are all exposed to the same germs. It's just that for some of us, our army is standing by ready to engage in battle while for others, they already are.

Below is a list of the top ten causes of death in the United States in order:

1) Heart disease
2) Cancer
3) Chronic lower respiratory disease
4) Stroke
5) Accidents
6) Alzheimer's disease
7) Diabetes
8) Influenza and pneumonia
9) Kidney disease
10) Suicide

Guess how many of these, according to the Centers for Disease Control and Prevention in 2011, are attributed chronic inflammation? Seven! Heart disease, cancer, chronic lower respiratory disease, stroke, Alzheimer's disease, diabetes, and kidney disease can all be directly linked chronic inflammation.

What can be considered a low intensity irritant? All of the foods I am trying to get you to stop eating in this book, which happen to be the same foods linked to intestinal permeability mentioned above. Other irritants can be alcohol, medications like non steroidal anti-inflammatory drugs (aspirin, ibuprofen, and naproxen), tobacco, and stress.

Note:

Non steroidal anti-inflammatory drugs (NSAIDs) have been linked to gastrointestinal damage (Hmmm), heart disease and stroke (Number one and number four from the above list). The evidence is so blatant that the Food and Drug Administration has pulled numerous prescription NSAIDs off the market and requires warning labels on the over the counter ones, with the exception of aspirin.

Food Baby

People who eat the way I eat tend to hang out together, especially online. A very common thing I have seen over the years is people posting pictures of their inflamed gut, most commonly called a food baby or gluten baby. These posts come from people who don't eat wheat but sometimes, whether intentional or not, get "glutened." This "baby" is irritation caused by gluten, which is the source of the Gliadin I mentioned earlier. For most of the people, including me, the swelling and irritation goes away after a couple days or so.

Now this reaction would be considered acute inflammation, but what if the person ate wheat again at their next meal or the next day and the next and the next? This would result in chronic inflammation.

Got that "itis?"

Chronic inflammation can also be attributed to any disease or condition that ends in "itis." Below are some of the most common ones:

- Rheumatoid arthritis
- Osteoarthritis
- Periodontitis
- Hashimoto's thyroiditis
- Sinusitis
- Ulcerative colitis

Guess what is commonly prescribed to people who suffer from arthritis? NSAIDs! Which can lead to chronic inflammation, the cause of arthritis! Basically, people are taking pills that could be making the very condition they are taking them for, worse.

The Bee Sting

Remember the bee sting I mentioned earlier? If you or anyone you know has ever been stung by a bee, then you may have seen how much swelling it caused. This is inflammation in action. Now, imagine your internal organs having the same reaction because of the irritants you consume.

I want you to keep in mind that you heart and lungs are protected by your ribcage. They are also separated from the rest of your internal organs by a wall of muscle know as the diaphragm. Your diaphragm basically lies horizontally right at the bottom of your rib cage. Right below your diaphragm are your liver and stomach. Now if these two organs swell up, where do you think they are going to go? Not up. You diaphragm prevents that. How about down? Nope, your other organs take up the rest of the space in your thoracic cavity. The only option is OUT! This is the part of your belly you can't seem to get rid of.

You may or may not have excess body fat but if you have a belly, especially right below your rib cage, I am willing to bet a big part of that is inflamed organs.

You can exercise and restrict your calories all you want but if you are still eating irritating foods, neither will reduce the inflammation in your gut. This is why so many of you go on diets or start strenuous workout routines and don't see results. If you do, chances are they are minor or temporary.

Diabetes

Diabetes is so common now that, according to a nurse friend of mine, when people are asked, "How is your blood sugar?" they are responding, "Oh not bad. It's around 200." Hello! This is **not** "not bad." This is double of what normal is. DOUBLE! Also, this same nurse tells me that when she asks patients if they have any conditions that she needs to know about they often respond with "no" even thought they have diabetes. This is a disease! It is so common though, that people seem to accept it. Let me tell you, it's not ok! Diabetes will guarantee you one of two things, an early death or a miserable last 10 to 20 years of your life.

When you eat a doughnut, the sugar and the flour cause your blood sugar levels to spike, almost immediately. This signals your pancreas to release insulin so it can do its job, which is to regulate your blood sugar levels by delivering the sugar to your muscles and liver in the form or glycogen. If these glycogen stores are full, the insulin carries the sugar to fat cells for storage making the fat cells larger and you fatter. If you eat another doughnut, or wash it down with a latte, this process continues. Taxing your pancreas like this may not be so bad on occasion but if it happens everyday, meal after meal, you are going to develop problems.

Problem 1: Your liver and muscles no longer respond to the insulin. They become resistant and tell insulin to bugger off. This is known as "Insulin Resistance" and can be an indicator of, or lead to, pre-diabetes.

Problem 2: Your pancreas says, screw it. After years of trying to regulate your blood sugar, your pancreas will eventually just call it quits. When this happens, congratulations, you're a diabetic.

Problem 3: High blood sugar, which can affect anything that relies on blood flow in order to work. These are some of the best parts of your body. These include your eyes, your kidneys, your heart, your feet, your brain and, for males, take a guess.

Diabetes is number 7 on this list of top ten causes of death in the United States mentioned above. The funny thing is, it leads to four other causes of death on that very same list. Number 1: Heart Disease, Number 4: Stroke, Number 6: Alzheimer's, and Number 9: Kidney Disease. Type

II diabetes is not something that should be taken as lightly as it is. The messed up part about it, it's completely preventable.

By law, I can't tell you that that going Primitive will cure any of the diseases I mention in this chapter but I can tell you the it can DRASTICALLY reduce chronic inflammation, the actual cause of the diseases listed in this chapter.

CLOSING THOUGHTS

Very few people are going to eat this way 100% of the time. Stuff happens. Chances are, you are going to eat some cheese after you give up dairy or you'll want to have some pancakes with maple syrup after you give up sugar. When this happens, know that you are **not** a bad person. In fact, you are a **strong** person battling against an entire society that tries it's damnedest to persuade you to eat crap food. Commercials, billboards, magazines, friends, family, and god know's who or what else are all trying to convince you that you are crazy for trying to eat this way. So, it's no wonder why we eventually fall off the wagon. Don't beat yourself up over it. It happens to the best of us.

When I decide to indulge, I try to plan it. Also, I eat the best of that thing I can get. If I'm going to eat pizza, I eat the best pizza I can find. There is a place in town here that has the best gluten free pizza I've had so far. President Obama has even eaten there. If I am going to eat a pastry, I do not eat the junk you can get at the convenience store. I'll drive to the other side of town to get the best cinnamon rolls on earth if I have to. My point is, if you are going to eat something that's not "Primitive," make it worth it.

Also, make it a special occasion. Do not eat this stuff at home and definitely don't keep it in the house. Once this starts to happen, you may end up finding yourself at square one. Going out for a slice of pumpkin pie is an occasional treat. Having a pie in the fridge is going to be the start of a new (or old) habit.

I have armed you with a lot of knowledge and a great process to achieve your goal. Just know that you are allowed to make it work for you. If you are an athlete and want to eat white rice for more energy, go for it. I'm not going to be mad at you. Also, if you fall off, know that you can always come back to the program.

If you are interested in some support for the program I encourage you to check out www.theprimitiveyou.com.

Best of luck,

Dave

THE NEXT STEP

Are you looking to lose weight? Well, if you follow the plan laid out in this book, you will. But, if you don't read my follow up book, Stop Working Out!, the weight will probably come back. In Stop Working Out! I address the issues with weight loss that are often overlooked with most weight loss plans. Click the image below for more info or to download it directly to your kindle.

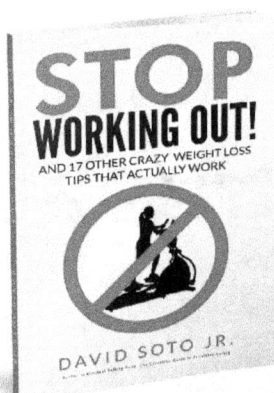

ABOUT THE AUTHOR

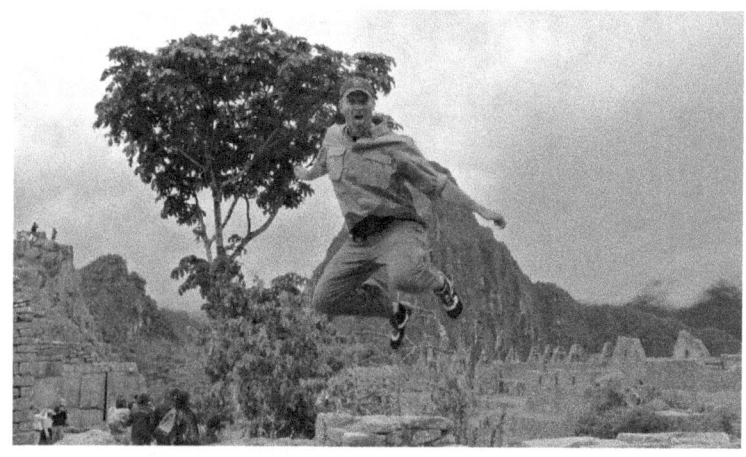

David was born in Gardena, California and spent most of his childhood in Los Angeles. In high school, his family moved to a small town in Missouri. At age 17, David joined the Air Force and spent the next 23 years toggling between active duty Air Force and the Missouri Air National Guard. In 2002 he was deployed under Operation Enduring Freedom and in 2004 he went to Iraq as a civilian contractor because his Air Guard Unit would not send him themselves.

Throughout the years, when not in uniform, David tried his best to fit into society. He got a job, went into debt to buy a house and a car, and tried to find a girl to marry and start a family with. None of these seemed to work out for him. Instead, he felt best on the road. At the age of 30, he sold most of his possessions, put his house up for rent, hit the road, and (more or less) hasn't stopped since.

Currently, David works with clients as a personal weight loss and life coach. He writes and speaks about how to regain your freedom through simplification. He calls it: Primitive Living. You can learn more about his philosophy at www.theprimitiveyou.com.